WRINKLE CREAM GUIDE FOR BEGINNERS

Anti-Aging Wrinkle Cream Recipes to Naturally Rejuvenate & Hydrate your Skin

SOFIE KING

Table of Contents

Introduction

I want to thank you and congratulate you for purchasing this book!

This book contains proven steps and strategies on how to create natural skin care products to prevent and minimize your wrinkles. You will be able to save money on great skin care without compromising on the results.

Thanks again for purchasing this book, I hope you enjoy it! Please take some time to stop by and LIKE our Facebook page:

https://www.facebook.com/joypublishing

With gratitude,

SOFIE KING

Chapter 1

How Wrinkles Form?

In order to understand how to take care of your skin better, you must understand how wrinkles and other signs of aging form. Many people think that wrinkles form due to dry skin, but this is a mistake. While dry skin can exacerbate the formation of wrinkles and can make them more visible, dry skin does not necessarily cause them. What happens is dry skin does not have enough of the natural skin oil or sebum whose purpose is to protect the skin from the elements like sun, cold and wind. Thus, those with dry skin can easily form wrinkles even at a young age.

Further, if someone already has wrinkles and has dry skin too, the lack of sebum causes the wrinkles to become more prominent. Sebum or other moisturizers can plump up the skin causing wrinkles to look less deep or prominent. This is why those with mature skin are encouraged to use rich or very emollient moisturizers. It might seem as if the moisturizer 'cures' the wrinkles, but they will soon be visible again once the moisture wears off or once that person washes her face.

Also, many think that only old people can get wrinkles. While this is true for most cases, some old folks can have youthful looking skin. Also, young people can get wrinkles if they do not properly take care of their skin. The signs of aging start to show by the age of 30, but this does not mean they have not started to accumulate as early as one's teenage years. If you spent most of your younger years under the sun without sun protection products or if you don't take care of your skin with proper nutrition or skin care products, the damage will accumulate deep in the skin's dermis layer and will show up by the time you reach your late 20s or early 30s. Those who spend their whole days under the sun since childhood might see signs of aging as early as their mid-20s.

What we must understand here is that skin damage slowly accumulates. If you spend only one day a year under the sun without sun protection products, your accumulated damage will be less compared to someone who spends every day under the sun.

Of course, unless you never go outside and never sit beside a clear window, and unless you live in a pristine environment with no hint of air or water pollution, you cannot escape from skin damage. Monks who live in dark monasteries can reach the age of 80 but still have the smooth and clear skin of a teenager. If living in the dark is not appealing to you, then rest assured that there are ways to prevent and minimize skin damage.

The skin accumulates damage due to UVA rays and free radicals in the environment. UVA rays or ultraviolet rays A are responsible for the majority of the signs of skin aging but most especially for the breakdown of collagen and elastin in the skin's dermis layer. These are the proteins necessary to keep the skin looking smooth, firm and bouncy.

While the body can replace damaged collagen, the natural aging process slows down the rejuvenating powers of the body. This is why a 20 year old who has experienced intense sun for a long period of time, e.g. a week's holiday at the beach, will have less damage than a 40 year old who has experienced the same.

It is also possible that the damage received on a daily basis is too much for the body to handle. A 20 year old who receives daily sun damage will probably have the same skin as a 40 year old who only receives sun damage in the form of his yearly beach trip.

UVAs can permeate even through clouds and thick but clear glass windows. Thick, tightly woven clothing can provide some protection but thin weaves will allow most of it to pass through. The other kind of ultraviolet ray, UVB, is responsible for tanning the skin. It does not cause as much damage to collagen and elastin but it can dry the skin and can contribute to an increased risk of developing skin cancer.

Moving on to free radicals, these are atoms or molecules with an unpaired electron in its outer shell. If you still remember your high school chemistry, you'll know that having an extra electron makes this atom or molecule unstable. It needs to join up with another atom or molecule from which it will 'steal' a proton. If it 'steals' protons from your skin cells, this will cause damage. While damage to one skin cell will not be significant, a lot of damage, especially if it accumulates over time, will result in an increase in wrinkles.

Free radicals are plentiful in polluted environments like cities or areas near factories. This is why people who live in these areas can look older than those who live in the country or in cleaner environments assuming they give their skin the same level of care. Free radicals can also enter the body through certain foods like junk food and excess sweets, but their effect will mostly be seen in other parts of the body like an impaired immune system and cancer of the internal organs. As far as the skin is concerned, most of the damage will come from air and water pollution when it comes into contact with the skin.

While free radicals can cause damage, it plays a small part in the formation of wrinkles. The sun still causes about 90% of the signs of aging with 10% caused by other factors. Thus, if someone lives in the country where the environment is clean but he is always out in the sun, he will have a lot of skin damage.

In addition to the sun and free radicals, we must include the destructive abilities of unhealthy habits like smoking, lack of proper nutrition and lack of sleep.

Smoking pours several poisons into the body which the body must try to remove if it does not want to die. The effort of cleansing the body of the poisons from cigarettes can tire it so much that it cannot focus on taking care of its various parts. This is why the immune system can weaken, the internal organs can become diseased and the skin becomes dull and sickly looking. If you are a young person whose body's rejuvenating powers are still at its peak, then your body can easily heal even if you smoke 2 packs a day, but only up to a certain point. By your mid-20s, the body might be too exhausted and slowly degenerate.

Regarding the lack of proper nutrition, the human body is an animal body and needs nourishment outside of itself. We need the various nutrients in their proper amounts to keep the body running. Even young people whose bodily functions are at their peak will soon break down if proper nutritional needs are not met.

Since the skin is part of the body, lack of nutrition will affect it. For example, vitamin A is necessary for the maintenance and repair of the skin. If your diet lacks it, your body might still have the ability to repair skin if you are still relatively young, but without the proper tools it will not do a very good job. To give an analogy, think of a skilled craftsman without the proper tools. He might be able to do the job but it will not be as good as when he has all the required tools.

Lastly, sleep is very important since this is the time when the body does its major repairs. Even if you are still young and eat properly, the lack of sleep does not give the body a chance to heal. Again, to give an analogy, this is like a skilled craftsman with the proper tools who is not given a break from work. Soon, tiredness will affect him and he will make mistakes that will affect the quality of his work.

Notice that there are several factors that cause skin damage and exacerbate it. You have to take all these things into consideration when determining how to prevent wrinkles. To summarize, here are the things that cause and exacerbate the signs of aging:

- UVA rays

- Free radicals

- Dry skin or the lack of sebum which acts as *some* protection against the sun, wind and cold.

- The body's lessened ability to regenerate itself which naturally happens due to aging. Generally speaking, the slowing down of the skin's ability to regenerate itself starts around the age of 30.

- Unhealthy habits like smoking, improper diet and lack of sleep.

These factors all contribute to the damaged collagen and elastin in the dermal layer of the skin. If the dermis is damaged, the epidermis follows the form of the damage. This shows up in the form of wrinkles.

Chapter 2

The Truth about Preventing Wrinkles

Now that we know what causes wrinkles, we can easily prevent it. Obviously, what we need to do is to avoid or minimize exposure to the causes listed above.

Since the sun causes 90% of skin damage, that is our number 1 concern. A variety of sun protection products exist in the market today to shield our skin from the UV rays, but most people don't know how to choose the best products. They also don't know how to properly use them.

In the first place, they choose a product according to the SPF (sun protection factor) number. That only indicates the amount of protection given against UVB rays. I am not saying that protecting yourself against UVB rays is bad, but as far as skin aging is concerned, you must focus on protecting yourself against UVA.

This is why it is more important to focus on the PA (protection against UVA) rating. You can know this according to the number of +'s indicated. PA+ gives you minimal protection and is best for those who only get about 10 minutes of sun. Those who are more exposed should look for PA++ or even PA+++.

In the second place, while people *do* apply sun protection, they do not apply enough. You need about 2 teaspoons of product for your whole face and neck and about 2 shot glassfuls for the whole body if you are going to expose most of your skin. If you are only going to expose your arms or hands, use a similar amount as you would for hand lotion.

You need to use these amounts to get the level of protection indicated in the package. If you don't then your SPF 15 might only be an SPF of 10 or 5. Also, don't skimp on sun protection even if you use make-up or moisturizers with SPF and PA. Since you don't use 2 teaspoons of these products on your face and neck, you are not using enough to provide adequate protection. The protection provided by these products is a good plus, but you must not solely depend on them.

Properly using sun protection products also means reapplying often. Ideally, you should reapply every 2 hours if you are under the sun, but if you have been sweating profusely or have been swimming, you should reapply immediately even if it has only been an hour. If you dislike reapplying throughout the day, you are better off using the highest level of protection you can find. Instead of 2 hours, you can get away with reapplying every 4 hours.

Now let us discuss the prevention of free radical damage. This can be avoided by applying topical skin care with antioxidants. The antioxidants protect the skin by attaching to the free radicals thus preventing them from attaching and damaging the skin cells.

The jury is still out regarding which antioxidant is best for the skin so don't worry too much about what to get. Instead, choose products according to your skin type and personal preference like fragrance, texture, packaging and the like.

You can also prevent free radical damage by eating your antioxidants. Increasing your intake of fresh fruits and vegetables, and other foods that are rich in antioxidants like tea, dark chocolate and red wine can all contribute to better skin. However, the difference between ingested and topical antioxidants is the latter can better protect the skin while the former will be directed to various parts of the body. After all, the body has several other organs it must take care of, but this is not to say that an increased intake of these good foods will not have an effect on the skin. As we have said, proper nutrition allows the body to function properly, including the repair of its damaged parts.

Regarding dry skin, as we have discussed previously, well-hydrated skin can better protect itself from the natural elements. We will discuss ways to hydrate the skin in the next chapter.

Regarding the body's lessened ability to regenerate itself, nothing can be done to prevent this, but something can be done to help the skin regenerate itself to minimize the effects of accumulated damage. We will discuss this further in chapter 4.

Lastly, when it comes to your unhealthy habits, it is your responsibility to take care of your body. If you smoke, stop. If you don't eat well, make an effort. If you don't sleep enough, rearrange your schedule to avoid too much work or make your bedroom more relaxing. If you are serious about taking care of your skin, you must become serious about taking care of your body. All the tips listed in this book will be for nothing if you still insist on your unhealthy habits.

Chapter 3

Recipes for Wrinkle Prevention

Here are some recipes for natural skin care products. They are a good substitute for commercially available products because they are cheaper in the long run. Also, you can tailor them according to your needs.

Before we discuss these recipes, we must mention some reminders when making products at home:

- Use a separate saucepan, mixers, bowls, etc. for your skin care products. You might need to use ingredients that are poisonous when ingested.

- Measure your ingredients well. Too much of an ingredient can cause irritation or will not result in a good product.

- Some ingredients are poisonous when inhaled. For safety reasons, use a mask when making these products.

- Use sterilized opaque glass containers for your finished products. You can sterilize them by pouring boiling water over them then leaving them to dry. Opaque glasses will help prevent their disintegration due to sunlight, but if you cannot find opaque glass containers, just keep your products in a dark place.

- If you live in a hot climate, it is best to store your natural products in the refrigerator, but make sure that no will suspect it for food. Label all products well and keep them out of children's reach.

- Buy ingredients from reputable sources. For example, make sure that you are buying fresh Shea or cocoa butter. Beeswax should be purified and free from bee bodies or traces of honey. Essential oils should be true oils and not artificial fragrance oils.

- If you have sensitive skin, always do a skin test before using any of these products. If you have extremely sensitive skin, it is best to stick to the commercially available products that have been tested for safety. Otherwise, those who are not so sensitive will generally not experience any irritation with the recipes listed in this book.

Sun Protection Cream

(This will give you SPF 20 and PA+, but you can add more zinc oxide to increase the level of protection. Doing this might make your cream leave a whitish cast that is especially obvious on dark skin. Experiment with the amount of zinc oxide that works best for you, but do not use less than 2 tablespoons for ½ cup of cream base.)

Ingredients:

- ¼ cup coconut, almond or jojoba oil (normal skin), or olive, argan or avocado oil (dry skin) or grape seed oil (oily skin)
- ¼ cup beeswax (normal or oily skin) or Shea or cocoa butter (dry skin)
- 2 tablespoons non-nano zinc oxide powder (do not inhale)

Procedure:

1. Melt the beeswax or Shea or cocoa butter in a saucepan.

2. Remove from the heat. Add the oil and mix well.

3. Add the zinc oxide and mix thoroughly.

4. Pour into your prepared container and allow to cool before using.

Antioxidant Toner

Ingredients:

- ½ cup strongly brewed green tea (use 1 tea bag in ½ cup of boiling water)
- 5 drops of green tea essential oil
  Optional: 2 drops of lemon, jasmine or lavender essential oil for fragrance

Procedure:

1. Once the tea is cooled, mix everything together in a glass bottle.

2. Use a cotton ball to apply. Shake well before every use.

Antioxidant Moisturizer

Ingredients:

- ¼ cup coconut, almond or jojoba oil (normal skin), or olive, argan or avocado oil (dry skin) or grape seed oil (oily skin)
- ¼ cup beeswax (normal or oily skin) or Shea or cocoa butter (dry skin)
- 10 drops of green tea essential oil
  Optional: 2 drops of lemon, jasmine or lavender essential oil for fragrance

Procedure:

Melt the beeswax or Shea or cocoa butter in a saucepan.

Remove from the heat. Add the oil and mix well.

Once it is well-mixed, add the essential oils and mix again.

Pour into your container and allow to cool before using.

Apply a pea sized amount all over the face and neck. If you used lavender essential oil, avoid applying near the eyes.

Basic Dry Skin Cream

(This can also be used for rough patches like elbows and knees.)

Ingredients:

- ¼ cup olive, argan or avocado oil
- ¼ cup Shea or cocoa butter

Procedure:

1. Melt the butter in a saucepan.

2. Remove from the heat and add the oil. Mix well.

3. Pour into your container and leave to cool.

Basic Dry Skin Facial Oil

(Facial oil is good for those who travel frequently. Since the oil is more emollient, you don't need much. A small amount will last you a long time. For extremely dry skin or during cold weather, apply the oil first then the cream. This oil can also be applied to dry hair and rough spots like elbows and knees.)

Ingredients:

- ¼ cup olive, argan, or avocado oil
- *Optional:* 2 drops of your choice of essential oil to add fragrance. Do not use lavender, peppermint or other similar scents if you wish to use this around your eye area.

Procedure:

1. Keep your oil in a bottle.

2. Add the essential oil and shake together to mix.

3. Use 1-2 drops of oil for moisturizing the whole face.

Rose Dry Skin Cream

(This has the natural feminine fragrance of roses. Do not use this if you are allergic to fragrance. Using fragranced products makes you look forward to using moisturizer. This is also a good choice for mature skin with deep wrinkles.)

Ingredients:

- 1 batch of basic dry skin cream
- 4 tablespoons of rosehip oil
- 5 drops of rose essential oil
  Optional: 2 drops of sandalwood essential oil (This will give your cream a more mature, sophisticated scent.)

Procedure:

1. Follow the steps in making the basic dry skin cream. Add the rosehip oil with the other oils.

2. After the rosehip oil is well-mixed, add the rose essential oil. Mix further then pour into your container.

Rose Dry Skin Facial Oil

Ingredients:

- 1 batch of basic dry skin facial oil
- 4 tablespoons rosehip oil
- 5 drops rose essential oil
  Optional: 2 drops of sandalwood essential oil

Procedure:

1. After making a batch of basic dry skin facial oil, add the other ingredients.

2. Shake well to mix.

Chapter 4

The Truth about 'Curing' Wrinkles

Now let us discuss what you have to do when you already have wrinkles. I have used the word 'cure' here but I only do this to prove a point about wrinkles. Once you have them, you cannot completely 'cure' them. What you can do is only to minimize their appearance, i.e. make them less deep. Thus, the truth about 'curing' wrinkles is this: it is impossible. The best way to keep your skin's youthful appearance is to prevent the signs of aging from showing up.

At this point you might say, 'But wait? What about those people with wrinkles who go through certain procedures and emerge looking youthful and fresh?'

Look at the before and after pictures closely. If the 'after' picture shows a person with an extremely youthful appearance, the 'before' picture likely shows a person without that much signs of skin aging, perhaps only a few shallow wrinkles around the eyes and mouth. The point here is you have to consider the starting point to understand how much improvement can be expected, and the answer will always be 'not 100%'.

Now you might think, 'but what about those who get a face lift?' The face lift stretches the skin so the wrinkles seem to smoothen, but that results in an unattractive 'tight faced' look. You have not actually cured the wrinkles but merely disguised them.

If this is the truth about 'curing' wrinkles, then what exactly can be done? 2 things can be done to 'cure' or minimize wrinkles: temporarily plumping the skin with moisturizer to disguise wrinkles, and forcing the skin to produce more collagen and elastin to make the wrinkles shallower. Now remember that since you cannot completely remove a wrinkle once it has formed, the collagen and elastin which certain skin care products can create will never be enough to bring your damaged skin back to its youthful glory, but at least the damage will be minimized.

First, let us discuss how to temporarily plump the skin. In chapter 1, we talked about how dry skin makes wrinkles more obvious because the skin is not plumped up. To give a rather obvious analogy, dry skin is like a raisin and adding moisturizer is like soaking that raisin in water. As the water gets into the raisin, it plumps up and its wrinkles become shallower.

To temporarily plump up the skin, you can use the dry skin cream or facial oil recipes described above or one of the commercially available products specifically made for dry skin. These products are extremely emollient and are designed to minimize water loss from the skin's cells. To increase the skin's water content, thus allowing it to look plumper, apply moisturizer on damp skin. In the middle of the day or whenever your skin feels dry, you can spritz some water on your face then apply more moisturizer.

You can do this even if you are wearing make-up, but you'll have to reapply more make-up since the moisturizer will dilute the colors. Just make sure that you only do this on a clean face, i.e. if you have been walking around a smoggy environment, you probably need to wash your face first instead of adding more moisturizer and make-up on top of that layer of dirt.

Second, let's consider how to permanently add more collagen and elastin to your skin. The only products that have been actually proven to significantly increase collagen and elastin are tretinoin and peptides. Tretinoin is more effective but can be very irritating if used daily. Peptides are less effective but are gentler to the skin. Those with sensitive skin can use a lower percentage of tretinoin and alternate it with peptides. Those with normal skin can probably use tretinoin every day.

While some products may advertise their ingredients as being clinically proven to do the same, this may only mean that they were shown to improve collagen and elastin in sample human skin cells in a laboratory but not necessarily in actual human skin.

You can buy skin care products with tretinoin or peptides from commercially available brands. Do not attempt to make your own. Besides, you will not be able to buy pure tretinoin or peptides as ingredients.

That said, there are still ways to increase collagen and elastin through natural beauty products like certain essential oils and plant oils. For example, rosehip oil is high in vitamin A and can give you similar effects as tretinoin which is also a form of vitamin A. Essential oils like lavender, sandalwood and patchouli can stimulate the capillaries in facial skin; thus bringing more blood to those areas that in turn means more nutrients.

However, their effects will not be as significant as tretinoin and peptides. You will probably need to wait a year of daily applications of rosehip oil to see the same results tretinoin can give in 4 months or peptides in 6. With regard to essential oils, they can only indirectly increase collagen and elastin by encouraging the body to bring more nutrients to the skin and thus give the cells what they need to repair themselves.

If you do not support this practice with proper nutrition and with adequate sleep, the increased blood brought to your facial skin will do nothing since it will not bring with it the skin's nutrients. You will also cancel out any good effects if you insist on the habit of smoking.

Another way to increase collagen and elastin is by regularly exfoliating the skin. By removing the top layer of the epidermis, you force the skin to reproduce more skin cells and repair itself. However, exfoliation will not make the skin produce the same amount of collagen and elastin as tretinoin and peptides will encourage it to.

Finally, the application of topical vitamin C can help to increase collagen and elastin production but only to a certain degree and not as much as the result of using tretinoin or peptides. Vitamin C is necessary in the production of these skin proteins so providing the skin with this nutrient encourages it to repair itself.

Chapter 5

Recipes for Deep Wrinkles

Though you cannot create tretinoin or peptide products on your own, you can still create products that stimulate collagen and elastin production even if only slightly. You can alternate between using tretinoin and/or peptides and essential oil moisturizers. Also, exfoliate your skin at least once a week for dry skin and twice a week for normal skin. Exfoliating will also minimize dark spots and reduce the dullness that is common in aging skin.

Essential Oil Wrinkle Reducing Cream

(This can be used at night while the antioxidant moisturizer can be used in the mornings before applying your sun protection product.)

Ingredients:

- ¼ cup coconut, almond or jojoba oil (normal skin), or olive, argan or avocado oil (dry skin) or grape seed oil (oily skin)
- ¼ cup beeswax (normal or oily skin) or shea or cocoa butter (dry skin)
- 10 drops of lavender, patchouli, sandalwood, chamomile or rose essential oil

Procedure:

1. Melt the beeswax or Shea or cocoa butter in a saucepan.

2. Remove from the heat and add the oil. Mix well.

3. Mix in the essential oil then pour into your container. Allow to cool before using.

Essential Oil Wrinkle Reducing Facial Oil

Ingredients:

- ¼ cup coconut, almond or jojoba oil (normal skin), or olive, argan or avocado oil (dry skin) or grape seed oil (oily skin)
- 5 drops of lavender, patchouli, sandalwood, chamomile or rose essential oil

Procedure:

1. Pour the oil into a glass bottle.

2. Add the essential oil and shake to mix well.

Facial Scrub

(Use this if you prefer physical exfoliation, i.e. using grainy substances, rather than acids to exfoliate your face.)

Ingredients:

- 1 tablespoon coconut, almond or jojoba oil (normal skin), or olive, argan or avocado oil (dry skin) or grape seed oil (oily skin)
- 1 teaspoon fine sugar, oatmeal or cornmeal (you need to experiment on what works best for your skin, but avoid salt for facial skin even if it is finely ground since it is too harsh.)

Procedure:

1. Mix everything together in a small bowl.

2. Apply this on your clean face with your fingertips. Use circular motions. Do not scrub one area of the face for longer than 2 seconds.

3. Exfoliate your face for 1 minute or longer but not more than 2 minutes.

4. If your skin becomes red or inflamed, you either pressed too hard, exfoliated too long or need to change your choice of grainy scrub.

Facial Exfoliating Mask

(This uses chemical exfoliation through the acids in the ingredients to dissolve the dead skin cells.)

Ingredients:

- 4 tablespoons of yoghurt
- 1 tablespoon fresh lemon juice
- 1 tablespoon crushed fresh strawberries

Procedure:

1. Combine everything in a bowl.

2. Apply to your clean face but avoid the eye area.

3. Leave on for 15-20 minutes, then wash off.

Yoghurt and Sugar Exfoliating Scrub and Mask

(This combines physical and chemical exfoliation.)

Ingredients:

- 4 tablespoons yoghurt
- 1 tablespoon fine sugar
  Optional: 1 teaspoon honey

Procedure:

1. Combine everything in a bowl and apply to your face.

2. Use your fingertips to scrub the sugar all over but avoid the eye area.

3. After a minute of scrubbing, leave the mask on for 15-20 minutes, then rinse it off.

Vitamin C Moisturizer

(Since vitamin C is an antioxidant, this can replace the antioxidant moisturizer described above. Keep this in an opaque container since light can oxidize vitamin C and render it useless.)

Ingredients:

- 1 teaspoon of crushed vitamin C tablets
- 2 ounces of distilled water in an opaque bottle
- ¼ cup coconut, almond or jojoba oil (normal skin), or olive, argan or avocado oil (dry skin) or grape seed oil (oily skin)
- ¼ cup beeswax (normal or oily skin) or shea or cocoa butter (dry skin)

Procedure:

1. Dissolve the crushed vitamin C in the water. Set aside.

2. Melt the beeswax or Shea or cocoa butter in a saucepan.

3. Remove from the heat then add the oil. Mix well.

4. When the mixture has slightly cooled, add the vitamin C water and quickly mix everything together.

5. Pour into your container.

6. Cover the container immediately even if the mixture is still warm. When using this, get a pea-sized amount then quickly cover the jar to avoid product oxidation. Keep this in the refrigerator.

Conclusion

Thank you again for purchasing this book!

I hope this book was able to help you to know how to prevent and minimize wrinkles with natural, homemade skin care products.

The next step is to try out the recipes listed here and see what works for you.

In addition, please remember to LIKE our Facebook page in order to find other resources and upcoming promotions:

https://www.facebook.com/joypublishing

With sincere thanks,

SOFIE KING

Preview of "Fast Hair Growth for Beginners: Natural Hair Growth Secrets and Hair Loss Cure for Growing Long and Fast Hair"

Chapter 1

Hair Growth Facts

What do you think of the state of your hair right now? Is it thick or thin? Is it treated or natural? Does it feel soft and smooth or brittle and dull? The current state of your hair will determine how fast and how long the strands can grow.

The truth is that human hair generally grows at the same rate, which is approximately half of a millimetre every day, which means that your hair becomes half an inch longer every month. The healthier and younger you are, the faster your hair can grow out. Apart from that, your genetics and hormones are additional natural factors that play a major role in hair growth. Other factors would be the hair treatments that you choose, the everyday hair care products that you use, your nutritional intake and even the condition of your scalp.

Since your goal is to have long and beautiful hair, you should aim to protect it from anything that will impede it from growing out at its normal rate. Likewise, you should "feed" it the right nutrients and make an extra effort to protect and take care of it to ensure that it will not be damaged as it continues to grow. After all, the only thing that is stopping your hair from growing fast is if it is harmed in some way.

How Hair Grows?

In order to understand the nature of hair growth, let us take a look at the three phases that describe this natural process: the anagen phase, the catagen phase, and the telogen phase.

The anagen phase is the moment when hair pushes itself out from the follicle. It is the time when the hair is in the middle of the growth process. When the hair slowly detaches itself from the follicle and "dies", this is the catagen phase. Finally, it would reach the telogen phase when it is pushed out from the follicle and is shed off by the body.

Of course, not all of the hair on the scalp go through the phases at the same time. As new strands of hair are produced each day, old strands are shed off. New hair replaces old hair every day, which makes it a cycle.

However, the moment when old hair is *not* replaced by new hair, then hair loss takes place. This is a problem that many people, both men and women, face. Since it is such a common issue, many companies have tried to come up with a cure-all that promises to promote hair growth and hair loss. But keep in mind that hair will not grow out fast and long within a few weeks. No such product can do that, and anything that claims that it can actually means they can help keep the hair stay strong as it continues to grow out naturally.

Fortunately, there are plenty of ways on how you can get the hair that you have always wanted. As we all know, each person's physiological makeup is different, which is why not all remedies and tips work for everyone.

Check out the full story of this book on Amazon

Or go to: http://amzn.to/1DeVBMK

One Last Thing...

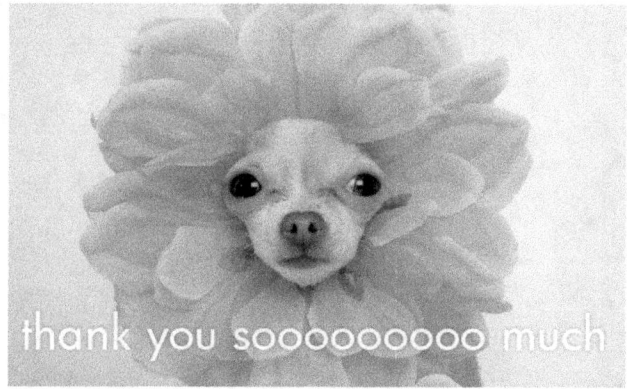

If you believe that this book is worth sharing, would you please take the time to let others know how it affected your life? If it turns out to make a difference in the lives of others, they will be forever grateful to you, as will I.